Managing Medical Costs

A Practical Guide to Reducing Healthcare and Prescription Expenses

By Oluchi Ike

Preface:

In today's world, the cost of healthcare has become a burden for many individuals and families. From skyrocketing insurance premiums to the high prices of prescription drugs, managing medical expenses can feel overwhelming and confusing. For those with chronic illnesses, complex health conditions, or those simply trying to maintain their well-being, navigating the healthcare system and understanding how to reduce costs has never been more critical.

This book was born out of a desire to empower people to take control of their healthcare expenses. Whether you're facing unexpected medical bills, struggling to afford necessary medications, or simply want to make more informed decisions about your health insurance options, this guide will provide you with the tools and strategies needed to manage your medical costs effectively.

We will break down the complexities of medical billing, explore options for lowering drug prices, and offer insights into government assistance programs that many people are unaware of. You'll also learn how to use online resources, telemedicine, and advocacy tools to ensure you're not paying more than you need to for healthcare services.

By the end of this book, you'll be equipped with practical knowledge and tips that will help you save money, navigate the healthcare system with confidence, and make informed choices for you and your family's medical needs. The goal is simple: to help you take charge of your healthcare expenses without sacrificing the quality of care you receive.

Table of Contents:

Chapter 4: Government and Non-Profit Assistance Programs

- Understanding Medicare and Medicaid: Eligibility and Benefits

- Other Government Programs That Help with Healthcare Costs

- Non-Profit Organizations: How They Can Help with Medical Bills

- Patient Assistance Programs from Pharmaceutical Companies

Chapter 5: Healthcare Savings Strategies

- How to Use Health Savings Accounts (HSAs) and Flexible Spending Accounts (FSAs)

- Preventive Care: Reducing Future Healthcare Costs

- Finding Affordable Healthcare Providers and Community Clinics

- Shopping for Cheaper Medical Procedures, Lab Tests, and Equipment

Chapter 6: Becoming Your Own Healthcare Advocate

- The Importance of Asking the Right Questions

- How to Dispute Medical Bills: Step-by-Step Guide

- When to Use a Medical Billing Advocate: How They Can Save You Money

- Legal Rights in Healthcare: Navigating Billing and Insurance Disputes

Chapter 7: Telemedicine and Digital Healthcare Solutions

- Telemedicine: A Cost-Effective Alternative to Traditional Visits

- Virtual Care vs. In-Person Care: Pros, Cons, and Cost Differences

- The Rise of Online Pharmacies: Convenience and Savings

Chapter 1: Introduction to Rising Medical Costs

Healthcare is an essential part of life, yet the costs associated with medical care have been steadily rising for decades. For many individuals and families, the financial burden of accessing basic healthcare services, medications, and treatments has become overwhelming. This chapter will provide an overview of the healthcare cost crisis, its impact on individuals and families, and how this book can help you navigate and reduce these expenses.

1.1 The Healthcare Cost Crisis

The cost of healthcare in the United States has reached unprecedented levels. According to data from the Centers for Medicare and Medicaid Services (CMS), national health expenditures are expected to exceed $6 trillion by 2028, which represents about 20% of the country's GDP. This increase has been driven by a combination of factors, including the rising cost of medical services, the price of prescription drugs, and administrative complexities within the healthcare system.

For many, accessing healthcare services has become prohibitively expensive. Even routine medical visits can result in substantial out-of-pocket expenses, and more significant treatments like surgeries, hospital stays, and ongoing therapies can push individuals into serious financial hardship. The problem isn't just limited to those without insurance—high-deductible health plans (HDHPs) and rising premiums mean even insured patients are facing greater costs before their coverage kicks in.

Prescription drug prices are also a major contributor to the healthcare cost crisis. Between 2014 and 2019, the cost of prescription medications increased by an average of 33%, far outpacing inflation. The price of insulin, for example, has become a symbol of this crisis, with many diabetics struggling to afford this essential medication despite having insurance.

This rising tide of costs has created a healthcare system that is unaffordable for millions of Americans. As a result, many people are delaying or avoiding necessary medical care, which can lead to worse health outcomes and even higher costs in the long term. Understanding the driving forces behind this crisis is the first step in learning how to manage and reduce these expenses.

1.2 The Impact on Individuals and Families

The financial strain of healthcare costs affects nearly every aspect of life for individuals and families. Medical bills are now a leading cause of personal bankruptcy in the United States, and many people are forced to make difficult choices between paying for healthcare and covering basic needs like housing, food, and education.

For those living with chronic illnesses, the costs are even higher. Individuals with conditions such as diabetes, heart disease, or cancer may face thousands of dollars in out-of-pocket expenses annually, even with insurance coverage. These costs can include doctor visits, ongoing treatments, specialized medications, and hospital stays. Over time, this financial burden can lead to stress, anxiety, and significant lifestyle changes.

Families with young children or aging parents face additional challenges. The cost of prenatal care, pediatric healthcare, and eldercare services, including nursing homes and assisted living facilities, can be exorbitant. Even a single medical emergency, such as an accident or sudden illness, can plunge a family into financial instability.

Beyond the direct financial costs, there are hidden consequences as well. High healthcare costs often discourage individuals from seeking preventive care, such as regular checkups, vaccinations, and screenings. This lack of preventive care can lead to more severe health issues down the road, further escalating costs and worsening overall well-being.

The emotional toll of managing medical expenses can be profound. The stress of dealing with mounting bills, insurance denials, and uncertainty about future care creates an environment of anxiety that can affect physical health, mental health, and relationships. The impact of rising healthcare costs is far-reaching, touching every aspect of daily life.

1.3 What This Book Will Help You Achieve

The good news is that while healthcare costs are high, there are practical strategies and resources that can help you navigate these challenges and reduce your expenses. The goal of this book is to equip you with the tools and knowledge to take control of your healthcare finances.

Throughout this book, you will learn:

- How to understand and negotiate medical bills to ensure you're paying a fair price for services.

- How to maximize your health insurance benefits, so you get the most value out of your coverage while minimizing out-of-pocket costs.

- Ways to lower prescription drug expenses, including the use of generic medications, discount programs, and patient assistance programs.

- Government and non-profit resources available to help with medical bills and drug costs, particularly for individuals with low incomes or those dealing with chronic conditions.

- How to use telemedicine and online services to access affordable care without sacrificing quality.

- Long-term savings strategies that can help you plan for future medical expenses, especially if you're managing a chronic illness or anticipating future healthcare needs.

This book is designed to be a practical guide, offering real-world advice and actionable steps to reduce the burden of healthcare expenses. Whether you're dealing with a specific medical issue or simply want to be better prepared for future healthcare costs, this book will help you make informed decisions and take proactive steps to manage your medical expenses more effectively.

The healthcare system may be complex and costly, but by becoming more informed and taking control of your medical decisions, you can significantly reduce your financial burden and ensure better health outcomes for you and your family.

This chapter sets the stage by acknowledging the scope of the healthcare cost problem and highlights how this book will guide readers through the process of managing these expenses. Would you like to dive deeper into any specific topics in future chapters?

Chapter 2: Understanding Medical Bills and Insurance

The healthcare system is notoriously complex, and one of the most confusing aspects for patients is understanding their medical bills and health insurance. The bewildering array of charges, fees, and insurance terms can leave you feeling lost, but this chapter will help demystify these concepts. By the end of this chapter, you'll know how to decode your medical bills, negotiate charges, and make informed decisions about your health insurance.

2.1 Decoding Your Medical Bills: Charges, Fees, and Hidden Costs

Medical bills are often full of jargon and itemized charges that are difficult to interpret. When you receive a bill after a hospital stay, doctor's visit, or procedure, it's important to carefully examine each line item. Here's a breakdown of some of the most common components found on medical bills:

- Itemized Charges: These include individual charges for every service, test, or procedure you received. From blood tests to imaging scans, hospitals and healthcare providers often charge separately for each service.

- Facility Fees: Hospitals and outpatient facilities often include a "facility fee" to cover the cost of using their equipment, operating rooms, and administrative support. These fees can be substantial and are frequently one of the largest items on a medical bill.

- Professional Fees: These refer to charges for the medical professionals involved in your care, such as doctors, surgeons, anesthesiologists, and other specialists. You may receive separate bills from each provider, even if they were part of the same procedure.

- Pharmacy Charges: If you received medications during your hospital stay or as part of a treatment, those costs will be listed separately, often with higher-than-usual prices compared to a retail pharmacy.

- Duplicate Charges: Always watch out for duplicate charges, where the same service or item appears more than once on your bill. This can happen by mistake and can inflate your final amount.

- Miscellaneous Fees: These can include everything from room charges to the use of medical supplies (like gloves and gowns) to fees for administrative tasks, such as medical record handling or paperwork.

Hidden Costs and Errors

In addition to understanding the basic categories on your medical bill, it's important to be aware of hidden costs and billing errors. Studies show that up to 80% of medical bills contain errors. Some common mistakes to watch for include:

- Incorrect Coding: Medical bills use special codes (such as CPT and ICD codes) to classify services and diagnoses. If the wrong code is used, it could lead to inflated costs or denial of insurance coverage.
- Unbundling: This occurs when services that should be billed as a single procedure are separated into individual charges, increasing the overall cost.
- Balance Billing: After your insurance pays its portion of the bill, some providers may try to bill you for the remaining balance, even though you shouldn't be responsible for these costs if you've met your deductible or out-of-pocket maximum.

Review your bills carefully, and don't hesitate to ask your provider or insurance company to explain any unclear or unfamiliar charges. Knowing how to read your bill is the first step toward controlling your healthcare costs.

2.2 How to Negotiate Medical Bills and Lower Charges

Negotiating medical bills can feel daunting, but it is often possible to reduce the amount you owe. Many healthcare providers are willing to work with patients on payment plans, discounts, or reductions, especially if you're uninsured or facing financial hardship. Here are some steps to take when negotiating medical bills:

1. Request an Itemized Bill: Always ask for an itemized bill to review the charges in detail. This will allow you to identify any errors or unnecessary charges.

2. Check for Errors: As mentioned in Section 2.1, billing errors are common. If you find any discrepancies, such as duplicate charges or services you didn't receive, contact the billing department and request a correction.

3. Compare Costs: Use online resources like Healthcare Bluebook or Fair Health Consumer to look up the average cost of the procedures or services you received. If your bill exceeds these average amounts, point this out to your provider and ask for a discount.

4. Negotiate Directly with the Provider: Call the billing department and explain your situation. Be polite but firm, and ask if they offer any discounts for uninsured patients, cash payments, or financial hardship. Many hospitals and doctors are willing to lower charges to help patients avoid financial distress.

5. Ask for a Payment Plan: If you're unable to pay the full amount upfront, ask if the provider offers a payment plan. Many hospitals and clinics have interest-free or low-interest plans that allow you to pay off the balance over time.

6. Use a Medical Billing Advocate: If negotiating on your own seems overwhelming, consider hiring a medical billing advocate. These professionals specialize in identifying errors and negotiating lower bills on behalf of patients.

7. Offer Cash Payments: Some providers offer significant discounts if you pay your bill in full with cash. This is especially helpful if your insurance didn't cover certain services, or if you don't have insurance at all.

Negotiating medical bills can save you hundreds, if not thousands, of dollars. The key is to be proactive, persistent, and informed about your rights as a patient.

2.3 Health Insurance Basics: Premiums, Deductibles, Co-Pays, and Networks

To understand how your medical costs are calculated and what you're responsible for, it's essential to understand the basic components of health insurance. Here are the key terms you need to know:

- Premium: The monthly amount you pay to your insurance company for coverage. Whether you use healthcare services or not, you're responsible for paying this amount regularly.

- Deductible: The amount you must pay out of pocket before your insurance begins to cover a portion of your medical expenses. For example, if your deductible is $1,500, you'll need to pay that amount before insurance kicks in.

- Co-Pay: A fixed amount you pay for a specific service, such as $30 for a doctor's visit or $10 for a prescription. Co-pays are usually due at the time of service.

- Coinsurance: This is the percentage of the medical cost you are responsible for after meeting your deductible. For example, if your coinsurance rate is 20%, you'll pay 20% of the total bill, while your insurance covers the remaining 80%.

- Out-of-Pocket Maximum: This is the most you will have to pay in a given year for covered services. Once you've reached this amount, your insurance will cover 100% of your medical costs for the rest of the year.

- Network: Health insurance plans often work with a specific network of doctors, hospitals, and pharmacies. In-network providers have agreed to offer services at lower, pre-negotiated rates, while out-of-network providers may charge more, leaving you with higher costs.

Understanding these terms is crucial to making informed decisions about your healthcare and how much you'll be expected to pay. The better you understand your health insurance plan, the more effectively you can use it to manage costs.

2.4 Choosing the Right Health Insurance Plan for Your Needs

Selecting the right health insurance plan can have a big impact on your healthcare costs. Here are some factors to consider when choosing a plan:

1. Understand Your Healthcare Needs: If you visit the doctor frequently or require ongoing care, you may want a plan with a lower deductible and higher premiums to reduce out-of-pocket costs. If you're generally healthy and don't anticipate needing much care, a high-deductible plan with lower premiums may save you money.

2. Compare Networks: Make sure your preferred doctors, hospitals, and pharmacies are in-network. Out-of-network care is often much more expensive, so sticking to in-network providers can save you significantly.

3. Check Prescription Coverage: If you take medications regularly, review the plan's drug formulary (the list of covered drugs) to ensure your prescriptions are covered.

Some plans offer better prescription coverage than others, so choose a plan that meets your medication needs.

4. Consider Your Financial Situation: Balancing premiums, deductibles, and co-pays is key. If you can afford higher premiums, a plan with lower out-of-pocket costs might be better. Conversely, if you want to keep monthly premiums low, be prepared for higher costs when you need care.

5. Take Advantage of Subsidies: If you qualify for government subsidies through the Affordable Care Act (ACA), you may be able to get more affordable health insurance. Check your eligibility for tax credits and cost-sharing reductions, which can significantly reduce your monthly premiums and out-of-pocket costs.

Choosing the right plan requires careful consideration of your healthcare needs, your financial situation, and the options available to you. Doing so can help you avoid unnecessary costs and ensure you have the coverage you need when it matters most.

By understanding how to decode medical bills, negotiate charges, and choose the right insurance plan, you're taking critical steps toward controlling your healthcare costs and ensuring financial security.

Chapter 3:

Prescription Drug Costs: What You Need to Know

Prescription drug prices in the U.S. have skyrocketed in recent years, placing a significant financial burden on individuals and families. From life-saving medications to common prescriptions, the rising cost of drugs has left many struggling to afford necessary treatments. In this chapter, we will explore why prescription drug prices continue to rise, discuss the differences between generic and brand-name medications, and provide actionable advice on how to find discounts, as well as lower-cost therapeutic alternatives.

3.1 The Rise in Prescription Drug Prices: What's Driving the Increase?

Prescription drug prices have been rising steadily over the past decade, far outpacing inflation. Many factors contribute to this increase, and understanding these dynamics can help you better navigate the pharmaceutical landscape.

One major factor driving up prices is patent protection. When pharmaceutical companies develop a new drug, they are granted exclusive rights through a patent, usually lasting 20 years. During this period, the company can set high prices without competition from generics. These high prices are often justified by the companies as necessary to recoup the cost of research and development (R&D), clinical trials, and bringing the drug to market. However, in many cases, the actual R&D costs are far lower than the revenues generated, leading to accusations of price gouging.

Another factor is limited competition. In certain cases, even after patents expire, few manufacturers enter the market to produce generic alternatives. This limited competition allows companies to maintain higher prices. Additionally, some drug makers employ strategies to extend patent life by making minor modifications to their drugs or creating combination medications, delaying the availability of cheaper generics.

Pharmacy Benefit Managers (PBMs) also play a significant role in shaping drug prices. PBMs act as intermediaries between insurers, pharmacies, and drug manufacturers, negotiating prices and rebates on behalf of insurance companies. While PBMs claim to save consumers money, critics argue that they often contribute to higher drug costs through complex rebate structures, lack of transparency, and by favoring high-cost brand-name drugs that offer larger rebates.

Finally, marketing and advertising costs drive up prices, especially for brand-name drugs. In the U.S., direct-to-consumer advertising of prescription drugs is legal, unlike in most other countries. Pharmaceutical companies spend billions each year promoting their medications, and those costs are ultimately passed down to consumers.

The result of these factors is an unsustainable situation where patients are forced to choose between essential medications and other basic needs. Understanding why prices are rising is crucial to finding ways to reduce your own drug costs.

3.2 Generic vs. Brand-Name Medications: Which is Right for You?

When faced with a high-cost prescription, many patients wonder whether switching to a generic version is a good option. To answer this question, it's important to understand the key differences between generic and brand-name medications, as well as their effectiveness.

Brand-name drugs are the original versions of a medication, developed and marketed by a specific pharmaceutical company. These drugs are often more expensive because they are under patent protection, meaning no other company can legally produce the same medication until the patent expires. Brand-name drugs typically have higher price tags due to the aforementioned R&D costs, marketing, and the monopoly held by the manufacturer.

Generic drugs, on the other hand, are chemically identical copies of brand-name drugs once the patent expires. They must contain the same active ingredients, be the same strength, dosage form, and route of administration as the brand-name version. Generic drugs undergo rigorous testing and must meet the same quality standards set by the U.S. Food and Drug Administration (FDA). The key difference is cost: generic medications are often 80-85% cheaper than their brand-name counterparts.

Is the quality the same?

Many patients worry that generics may be less effective than brand-name drugs, but this is not the case. The FDA ensures that generics work in the same way and provide the same clinical benefit as their brand-name counterparts. The inactive ingredients (such as fillers or coloring agents) may differ slightly, but these differences do not affect how the medication works.

When should you choose a brand-name drug?

There are a few situations where your doctor might recommend sticking with a brand-name drug, such as:

- Narrow Therapeutic Index (NTI) drugs: These are medications where even small differences in the dose or blood concentration can cause serious health problems. In such cases, doctors might prefer the brand-name version to ensure consistency.
- Allergies to inactive ingredients: If you have a known allergy to one of the inactive ingredients in a generic drug, you may need to stick with the brand-name version.

However, in most cases, choosing a generic drug can save you a significant amount of money without compromising your health.

3.3 Finding Prescription Discounts: Coupons, Cards, and Programs

Prescription costs can be overwhelming, but there are several ways to find discounts and lower the price of your medications. By taking advantage of coupons, discount cards, and assistance programs, you can often reduce your out-of-pocket costs dramatically.

Manufacturer Coupons and Patient Assistance Programs (PAPs)

Many pharmaceutical companies offer manufacturer coupons or patient assistance programs to help patients afford brand-name medications. These programs are especially helpful for those who are uninsured or underinsured, and they can sometimes provide free or discounted medications. You can often find these coupons on the drug manufacturer's website, through your doctor, or by asking your pharmacist.

For patients with low incomes or those who meet certain eligibility requirements, some manufacturers offer Patient Assistance Programs (PAPs), which can provide medications at no cost or at a steep discount.

Prescription Discount Cards

Various companies and non-profit organizations offer prescription discount cards that can be used to save money on medications. These cards, such as GoodRx, RxSaver, and SingleCare, are free to use and can help you find the lowest price available at local pharmacies. When you enter the name of your prescription on their websites, you'll get a comparison of prices at different pharmacies in your area. Simply present the card at the pharmacy, and you may pay much less than the retail price, even if you have insurance.

Pharmacy Discount Programs

Some pharmacies offer their own discount programs for certain medications, especially generic drugs. Large retailers like Walmart, CVS, and Walgreens have lists of medications available at low prices (sometimes as little as $4 for a 30-day supply). These programs often don't require insurance, making them accessible to anyone in need.

By combining manufacturer coupons, patient assistance programs, and prescription discount cards, you can often significantly reduce your prescription costs. Always ask your pharmacist if there are any discounts available and be proactive in searching for the best deals.

3.4 Exploring Therapeutic Alternatives: Lower-Cost Medications

Another strategy for lowering prescription costs is to explore therapeutic alternatives. These are medications that may not be identical to your prescribed drug but work in similar ways to treat the same condition.

For example, if your doctor prescribes a high-cost cholesterol-lowering medication, you might ask about switching to a less expensive statin or another drug class that has a similar effect. In many cases, older medications that have been on the market for longer are just as effective as newer, more expensive options.

Some steps to take when discussing therapeutic alternatives with your doctor:

1. Ask about lower-cost options: Be upfront with your doctor about the cost of your medication. They may be able to prescribe a less expensive drug that works just as well.
2. Check if a different dosage or form is cheaper: Sometimes, switching from a capsule to a tablet or adjusting the dosage can lower the cost.
3. Consult with a pharmacist: Pharmacists are often aware of therapeutic alternatives and can work with your doctor to suggest lower-cost medications.

By exploring therapeutic alternatives, you can often find equally effective treatments at a fraction of the cost.

Prescription drug costs don't have to break the bank. By understanding what drives the prices, choosing generic medications when appropriate, utilizing discounts, and considering therapeutic alternatives, you can take control of your healthcare expenses and make informed, cost-effective decisions.

Chapter 4:

Government and Non-Profit Assistance Programs

Healthcare costs continue to rise, leaving many individuals and families grappling with high medical and prescription bills. Fortunately, there are various government programs and non-profit organizations designed to provide assistance to those in need. Whether you're eligible for Medicare, Medicaid, or other government aid, or you're looking for non-profit resources, there are options that can help ease the financial burden. This chapter will guide you through the key programs available, including Medicare and Medicaid, other government initiatives, non-profit organizations, and patient assistance programs offered by pharmaceutical companies.

4.1 Understanding Medicare and Medicaid: Eligibility and Benefits

Medicare and Medicaid are two major government programs in the U.S. that offer healthcare assistance to different populations. While both are vital in providing financial relief for medical costs, they serve distinct groups and have unique eligibility requirements and benefits.

Medicare

Medicare is a federal health insurance program primarily for people aged 65 and older, although younger individuals with certain disabilities or conditions like End-Stage Renal Disease (ESRD) may also qualify. Medicare is divided into four parts, each covering different types of healthcare services:

➢ Part A (Hospital Insurance): Covers inpatient hospital stays, skilled nursing facilities, hospice care, and some home healthcare. Most people don't pay a premium for Part A if they or their spouse paid Medicare taxes for a certain period.

➢ Part B (Medical Insurance): Covers outpatient services, doctor visits, preventive care, and medical supplies. Part B requires a monthly premium, which varies based on income.

➢ Part C (Medicare Advantage): A private insurance alternative to Original Medicare that bundles Parts A, B, and often D into one plan. These plans may offer additional benefits like vision, dental, and hearing care.

➢ Part D (Prescription Drug Coverage): Helps cover the cost of prescription medications. Plans are offered through private insurers and involve an additional monthly premium.

Medicaid

Medicaid, on the other hand, is a joint federal and state program that provides health coverage for low-income individuals and families. Eligibility for Medicaid is determined by income level, family size, and other factors like disability status or pregnancy. The federal government sets broad guidelines, but each state administers its own Medicaid program with varying rules and benefits. Some states have expanded Medicaid under the Affordable Care Act (ACA), allowing more people to qualify based on income alone.

Eligibility and Enrollment

To qualify for Medicare, you must either be 65 or older, have a qualifying disability, or meet certain health criteria (such as ESRD). Most people are automatically enrolled in Medicare Part A and Part B when they turn 65 if they're already receiving Social Security benefits. However, you need to enroll yourself if you aren't automatically enrolled.

Medicaid eligibility varies by state, but it generally covers low-income individuals, pregnant women, children, seniors, and people with disabilities. If you qualify for Medicaid, you can enroll at any time, and there are no premiums or deductibles for most services, although some states may charge small co-pays.

Both programs provide essential coverage, but it's important to review your options and understand the benefits and potential out-of-pocket costs associated with each. Additionally, some individuals may qualify for dual eligibility, meaning they can receive both Medicare and Medicaid, which can significantly reduce healthcare expenses.

4.2 Other Government Programs That Help with Healthcare Costs

In addition to Medicare and Medicaid, there are several other government programs designed to help reduce healthcare and prescription costs for qualifying individuals. These programs can provide crucial financial relief, especially for those who don't meet Medicare or Medicaid eligibility or need additional assistance.

Children's Health Insurance Program (CHIP)

CHIP provides health insurance to children in low-income families who do not qualify for Medicaid but cannot afford private insurance. CHIP covers a range of healthcare services, including routine check-ups, immunizations, prescriptions, and dental care. Like Medicaid, CHIP is administered by states with federal guidelines, and eligibility varies based on income and family size.

Affordable Care Act (ACA) Subsidies

Under the Affordable Care Act, low- and middle-income individuals and families who purchase health insurance through the Health Insurance Marketplace may qualify for premium tax credits or subsidies to help reduce the cost of monthly premiums. Additionally, the ACA introduced Cost Sharing Reductions (CSRs), which lower out-of-pocket costs like deductibles and co-pays for qualifying individuals who select Silver-level plans.

Veterans Health Administration (VHA)

Veterans of the U.S. Armed Forces may be eligible for healthcare services through the Veterans Health Administration (VHA), which provides comprehensive medical care, including preventive, diagnostic, and treatment services. The VHA operates a network of hospitals, outpatient clinics, and long-term care facilities. Veterans who qualify for the VHA may pay little to no cost for healthcare, depending on their service history, income, and other factors.

State Pharmaceutical Assistance Programs (SPAPs)

Some states offer State Pharmaceutical Assistance Programs (SPAPs) to help residents cover the cost of prescription medications, especially for those on Medicare. These programs vary from state to state and may help cover Part D premiums, co-pays, and other drug-related costs.

Each of these programs offers valuable support for specific populations. If you qualify for any of them, enrolling can provide significant financial relief and access to necessary healthcare services.

4.3 Non-Profit Organizations: How They Can Help with Medical Bills

Non-profit organizations can also play a critical role in helping individuals and families manage high medical bills. These organizations often provide financial aid, access to low-cost healthcare, or assistance in negotiating bills with healthcare providers.

HealthWell Foundation

The HealthWell Foundation helps underinsured individuals cover the cost of prescriptions, co-pays, deductibles, and insurance premiums for specific medical conditions. Patients can apply for assistance directly through their website.

Patient Advocate Foundation (PAF)

The Patient Advocate Foundation offers financial aid to patients with chronic or life-threatening illnesses. Their Co-Pay Relief Program helps eligible patients cover co-payments required by their insurance, and their Case Management Program provides assistance with insurance disputes, job retention issues related to illness, and medical debt crisis intervention.

NeedyMeds

NeedyMeds is an online resource that helps people find programs to reduce their medication costs. The organization provides information on patient assistance programs, disease-specific assistance, and discounted medical services. NeedyMeds also offers a free drug discount card that can be used at participating pharmacies to save on prescription drugs.

The Assistance Fund (TAF)

The Assistance Fund helps individuals with serious or chronic conditions cover the cost of their healthcare, including medications and insurance premiums. TAF provides financial support to patients who meet income criteria and have a confirmed diagnosis of a covered disease.

Non-profits like these can make a significant difference, especially when dealing with overwhelming medical bills. Don't hesitate to reach out to these organizations if you need help; they exist to support people in challenging situations.

4.4 Patient Assistance Programs from Pharmaceutical Companies

In addition to non-profit organizations, many pharmaceutical companies offer Patient Assistance Programs (PAPs) to provide discounted or free medications to patients who cannot afford them. These programs are typically designed for uninsured or underinsured patients and are a valuable resource for those struggling with high prescription costs.

How Do Patient Assistance Programs Work?

Pharmaceutical companies set up PAPs to help patients access their medications at little to no cost. Each program has its own eligibility criteria, which may include income limits, lack of insurance, or inadequate coverage for the prescribed medication. Some PAPs provide free medications, while others offer significant discounts.

To apply for a PAP, patients typically need to:

1. Obtain an application form from the pharmaceutical company's website.
2. Provide proof of income and other documentation to demonstrate financial need.
3. Have their doctor complete a section of the application to confirm the need for the medication.
4. Submit the completed application for review.

Once approved, patients may receive their medications directly from the manufacturer or through a participating pharmacy.

Examples of Pharmaceutical Companies with PAPs

- Pfizer RxPathways: Offers financial assistance for Pfizer medications, including free drugs for those who qualify.
- Lilly Cares: Provides Eli Lilly medications at no cost to eligible patients.
- Sanofi Patient Connection: Assists patients with accessing Sanofi medications for free or at a reduced cost.

By taking advantage of these programs, patients can significantly reduce the financial burden of prescription drug costs. If you're having trouble affording your medication, ask your healthcare provider or pharmacist about available PAPs, or research them directly on pharmaceutical company websites.

Government and non-profit programs offer a lifeline to those burdened by high healthcare costs. By understanding and utilizing Medicare, Medicaid, other government initiatives, non-profit support, and patient assistance programs, you can alleviate some of the financial pressures associated with medical expenses.

Chapter 5: Healthcare Savings Strategies

Healthcare costs can feel overwhelming, but there are several strategies you can use to save money while ensuring you receive the necessary care. This chapter will focus on how to maximize savings through Health Savings Accounts (HSAs) and Flexible Spending Accounts (FSAs), the importance of preventive care, ways to find affordable healthcare providers and community clinics, and tips for shopping around for cheaper medical procedures, lab tests, and equipment. By adopting these strategies, you can take control of your healthcare expenses and avoid unnecessary financial strain.

5.1 How to Use Health Savings Accounts (HSAs) and Flexible Spending Accounts (FSAs)

Health Savings Accounts (HSAs) and Flexible Spending Accounts (FSAs) are powerful tools that allow you to save money on medical expenses by using pre-tax dollars. Both accounts help reduce the cost of healthcare by setting aside funds to pay for out-of-pocket medical expenses, but they operate differently, and understanding how each works can significantly boost your savings.

Health Savings Accounts (HSAs)

HSAs are available to individuals enrolled in high-deductible health plans (HDHPs). These accounts allow you to contribute pre-tax dollars to pay for qualified medical expenses, such as doctor visits, prescriptions, and even certain over-the-counter medications. One of the key benefits of HSAs is that the money you contribute rolls over year to year, so you don't lose the funds if you don't spend them within a certain timeframe. Additionally, HSAs offer a triple tax advantage:

1. Contributions are tax-deductible or made with pre-tax income.
2. The money grows tax-free if invested.
3. Withdrawals used for qualified medical expenses are also tax-free.

HSAs can be an excellent way to save for future medical expenses, especially for those who don't expect to use much healthcare in the short term. Another benefit is that after age 65, you can withdraw funds from your HSA for non-medical expenses without penalty (although you will pay income taxes on those withdrawals, similar to a traditional IRA).

Flexible Spending Accounts (FSAs)

FSAs are employer-sponsored accounts that also allow you to use pre-tax dollars for medical expenses. Unlike HSAs, FSAs are not tied to high-deductible health plans, and anyone with access to an employer-sponsored FSA can participate. FSAs have some important differences to consider:

- Use-it-or-lose-it rule: Generally, FSAs are subject to a "use-it-or-lose-it" rule, meaning any money left in the account at the end of the year is forfeited. Some employers may offer a grace period or allow you to roll over a small amount, but this varies.

- Lower contribution limits: FSAs typically have lower contribution limits than HSAs.

- Employer-provided: Unlike HSAs, you can only access an FSA through your employer, and you lose access if you change jobs or are laid off.

Both HSAs and FSAs provide significant tax advantages and can help you save on healthcare expenses, but it's essential to plan your contributions carefully, especially with FSAs, to avoid losing unused funds.

5.2 Preventive Care: Reducing Future Healthcare Costs

Preventive care is one of the most effective ways to reduce future healthcare costs. By focusing on early detection and regular check-ups, you can catch health issues before they become more serious — and more expensive to treat. Many health insurance plans cover preventive services at no cost to you, making it easier to prioritize your health without worrying about additional expenses.

What is Preventive Care?

Preventive care includes services like annual physicals, screenings, vaccinations, and health counseling that are aimed at preventing illness or detecting health conditions early. Examples include:

- Routine screenings: Mammograms, colonoscopies, and cholesterol checks help detect conditions like cancer or heart disease early.
- Vaccinations: Flu shots, pneumonia vaccines, and other immunizations protect against serious illnesses.
- Wellness visits: Annual physicals allow your doctor to monitor your overall health and catch potential problems early.
- Health counseling: Counseling on topics such as weight management, smoking cessation, and mental health can help you adopt healthier behaviors and reduce your risk of developing chronic conditions.

How Preventive Care Saves Money

Catching health issues early can save you money in the long run. Treating conditions like high blood pressure, diabetes, or high cholesterol early on can prevent costly complications such as heart attacks, strokes, or kidney failure. Preventive care can also help you avoid emergency room visits and hospitalizations, which are much more expensive than routine check-ups.

Additionally, many health insurance plans, including those through the Affordable Care Act, cover preventive care services at no out-of-pocket cost, meaning you can access these essential services without worrying about co-pays or deductibles.

5.3 Finding Affordable Healthcare Providers and Community Clinics

Accessing affordable healthcare is a major concern for many individuals, especially those without insurance or with high deductibles. Fortunately, there are ways to find healthcare providers and clinics that offer services at lower costs.

Community Health Centers and Clinics

Community health centers provide comprehensive medical services at reduced costs, often on a sliding fee scale based on your income. These clinics are a vital resource for individuals and families who may not have access to affordable healthcare otherwise. Services typically offered include primary care, dental care, mental health services, and preventive care like vaccinations and screenings.

Some clinics even offer specialized care, such as women's health services, prenatal care, and chronic disease management. These centers often partner with government programs like Medicaid and CHIP, ensuring that low-income patients receive the care they need.

Retail Clinics and Urgent Care Centers

Retail clinics, often located in pharmacies or supermarkets, provide affordable care for minor health issues, such as flu shots, infections, or minor injuries. These clinics are usually less expensive than a visit to a doctor's office or an urgent care center, and they often have transparent pricing so you know the cost upfront.

Urgent care centers can also be a more affordable option compared to emergency room visits, especially for non-life-threatening conditions. While they tend to cost more than retail clinics, they are still significantly cheaper than the ER and can treat issues like sprains, cuts, or minor fractures.

Telehealth Services

Telehealth services have become increasingly popular, providing patients with access to healthcare professionals from the comfort of their homes. Telehealth appointments are often more affordable than in-person visits, and many insurance plans now cover telehealth services. Telemedicine is particularly useful for managing chronic conditions, getting quick advice on minor ailments, or following up with a healthcare provider without the need for a physical visit.

By exploring these lower-cost options, you can still receive high-quality healthcare without the financial burden that often accompanies traditional doctor visits or hospital stays.

5.4 Shopping for Cheaper Medical Procedures, Lab Tests, and Equipment

Medical procedures, lab tests, and equipment can come with hefty price tags, but with some research and comparison shopping, you can often find more affordable options without sacrificing quality.

Medical Procedures and Surgeries

The cost of medical procedures can vary dramatically depending on the provider and location. For example, a knee replacement surgery could cost $20,000 at one hospital and $50,000 at another, even within the same city. Websites like Healthcare Bluebook and Fair Health allow you to compare the cost of procedures in your area, giving you the information you need to choose the most affordable option.

You can also consider medical tourism for certain procedures. Some countries, like Mexico, India, and Thailand, offer high-quality medical care at a fraction of the cost in the U.S. However, medical tourism requires careful research to ensure you're choosing a reputable facility and understanding the risks involved.

Lab Tests

Lab tests, such as blood work, X-rays, or MRIs, can also vary in price depending on where you go. Independent labs and imaging centers often charge much less than hospital-based facilities for the same tests. You can ask your doctor for a referral to an independent lab, or you can use websites like LabFinder to compare prices and book tests directly.

Medical Equipment

Whether you need crutches, a wheelchair, or home oxygen equipment, medical devices can quickly add up in cost. Shopping around for used or refurbished equipment can save you money. Many organizations and websites offer gently used medical devices at a fraction of the cost of new ones. Additionally, some insurance plans, including Medicare, may cover part of the cost of necessary medical equipment if prescribed by your doctor.

By taking advantage of savings strategies like using HSAs and FSAs, prioritizing preventive care, finding affordable healthcare providers, and shopping around for medical procedures and equipment, you can significantly reduce your healthcare costs while still receiving the care you need. These practical steps empower you to take control of your healthcare finances and protect yourself from unexpected expenses.

Chapter 6: Becoming Your Own Healthcare Advocate

Healthcare can be daunting, especially when it comes to understanding medical bills, insurance policies, and navigating the complex medical system. Many individuals feel overwhelmed by the rising costs and lack of transparency, which can make it difficult to make informed decisions. This chapter is about empowering you to take control of your healthcare by becoming your own advocate. By learning how to ask the right questions, dispute medical bills, leverage the help of medical billing advocates, and understand your legal rights, you can significantly reduce costs and ensure you get the care you deserve without unnecessary financial strain.

6.1 The Importance of Asking the Right Questions

When dealing with doctors, hospitals, and insurance companies, asking the right questions is critical to ensuring that you receive both the best care and the most accurate billing. Many people feel intimidated or rushed in healthcare settings, leading them to accept medical advice and costs without fully understanding them. Taking a proactive role in your healthcare by asking the right questions can help you avoid unnecessary procedures, inflated charges, and confusion about insurance coverage.

Questions to Ask Your Doctor

When receiving treatment, don't hesitate to ask your healthcare provider about the costs and necessity of recommended procedures or tests. Some key questions include:

- Is this procedure or test necessary? Doctors sometimes recommend tests that may not be urgent or essential. Clarifying the need can help avoid unnecessary expenses.
- Are there alternatives? There may be less expensive alternatives to certain treatments, such as generic drugs instead of brand-name medications or outpatient surgery instead of a hospital stay.
- What are the costs of this treatment? Many patients assume their doctor knows what procedures will cost, but that's not always the case. Asking this question prompts providers to check the cost, ensuring there are no surprises.

Questions to Ask the Billing Department

Before undergoing any procedure, it's also essential to ask your hospital or clinic's billing department for a detailed cost breakdown. Some important questions include:

- What is the total estimated cost of the procedure? Understanding the full cost upfront allows you to budget and negotiate more effectively.
- Does my insurance cover this procedure? Confirming with both your provider and insurer that the procedure is covered can help avoid unexpected out-of-pocket expenses.

- Are there any discounts for paying in cash or upfront? Some providers offer discounts if you pay in full or without involving insurance.

Asking these questions empowers you to make more informed decisions, and it ensures transparency in both your treatment and the associated costs.

6.2 How to Dispute Medical Bills: Step-by-Step Guide

Even with careful planning, medical bills can sometimes contain errors, overcharges, or surprise fees. Disputing medical bills may seem intimidating, but it can lead to significant savings if done correctly. Here's a step-by-step guide to disputing your medical bills effectively:

Step 1: Review Your Bill in Detail

Before disputing any charges, thoroughly review your medical bill. Look for unfamiliar charges, duplicate items, or procedures that you didn't receive. Request an itemized bill from the provider's billing department, which breaks down each charge in detail. Compare the bill with your insurance explanation of benefits (EOB) to ensure that what your provider charged matches what your insurance processed.

Step 2: Verify with Your Insurance Company

If a charge seems incorrect, contact your insurance company to verify the details. Sometimes insurance denies claims or processes them incorrectly, which can result in higher bills. Ask your insurer why a particular claim was denied or partially covered, and request that they reprocess the claim if necessary.

Step 3: Contact the Healthcare Provider's Billing Department

Once you've reviewed the bill and spoken with your insurance company, reach out to the billing department of the healthcare provider. Politely explain the discrepancies or overcharges you've identified and request a correction. Be specific about what items you believe are incorrect, and provide any supporting documents, such as your EOB or medical records, to back up your claim.

Step 4: Negotiate a Lower Bill

If the charges on the bill are legitimate but the cost is overwhelming, don't hesitate to negotiate. Many hospitals and providers are willing to reduce charges or offer payment plans. If you can pay a portion of the bill upfront, you may be able to negotiate a discount for doing so.

Step 5: Follow Up in Writing

After your phone calls, send a formal letter to both the provider and your insurance company detailing your dispute. Include all relevant documents and request confirmation of the correction in writing. Keeping a paper trail is crucial in case you need to escalate the dispute further.

By following these steps, you can avoid paying more than you should and reduce the financial burden of medical expenses.

6.3 When to Use a Medical Billing Advocate: How They Can Save You Money

In some cases, disputing medical bills can be complex, especially when dealing with high-cost procedures or multiple bills. If you're struggling to resolve issues on your own, hiring a medical billing advocate can be a worthwhile investment.

What is a Medical Billing Advocate?

A medical billing advocate is a professional who specializes in reviewing and negotiating medical bills on behalf of patients. They have in-depth knowledge of medical coding, insurance policies, and hospital billing practices, making them highly effective at identifying errors and overcharges. In some cases, they can even negotiate lower rates with healthcare providers.

How They Can Help

Medical billing advocates offer several services that can save you time and money:

- Identifying billing errors: They can spot mistakes like duplicate charges, incorrect billing codes, or services that were never rendered.

- Negotiating with providers: Advocates are skilled negotiators who can work with hospitals and doctors to lower your bill, often securing significant discounts.
- Managing insurance claims: If your insurance company has denied a claim or processed it incorrectly, a billing advocate can help file appeals and ensure you receive the coverage you're entitled to.
- Setting up payment plans: In cases where bills can't be reduced, advocates can help set up manageable payment plans, often with no interest or reduced rates.

When to Use One

While medical billing advocates charge a fee for their services, the savings they generate often far outweigh the cost. Consider hiring one if:

- You have a large or complicated medical bill that you don't fully understand.
- Your attempts to resolve billing errors have been unsuccessful.
- You're overwhelmed by medical debt and need help negotiating payment terms.

Many advocates work on a contingency basis, meaning they only get paid if they successfully reduce your bill, making it a low-risk option for substantial savings.

6.4 Legal Rights in Healthcare: Navigating Billing and Insurance Disputes

Understanding your legal rights is essential when it comes to disputing medical bills or dealing with insurance companies. The U.S. healthcare system is regulated by federal and state laws that protect patients from unfair billing practices, and knowing these rights can empower you to take action when necessary.

The No Surprises Act

The No Surprises Act, which went into effect in 2022, protects patients from surprise medical bills for emergency services, non-emergency services at in-network hospitals, and air ambulance services. Under this law, patients are only responsible for their in-network co-pay, deductible, or co-insurance for these services, even if the provider is out-of-network. If you receive a surprise bill for any of these services, you have the legal right to dispute the charge.

The Affordable Care Act (ACA) Protections

The ACA provides several protections that impact billing and insurance disputes, including:

- Free preventive care: Insurance companies are required to cover preventive services without charging a co-pay or deductible.
- Right to appeal: If your insurance company denies coverage, you have the right to file an appeal. If the appeal is denied, you can request an independent external review.
- Protections against lifetime and annual limits: Insurance companies are no longer allowed to impose lifetime or annual limits on essential health benefits.

State Laws

Many states have additional protections in place that regulate medical billing practices. Some states, for example, have laws that cap the amount hospitals can charge uninsured patients, ensuring they are billed at the same rate as insurance companies. Research your state's specific laws to see what additional rights you may have.

By becoming your own healthcare advocate, asking the right questions, disputing bills when necessary, leveraging medical billing advocates, and understanding your legal rights, you can significantly reduce your medical costs and protect yourself from financial hardship. In the complex world of healthcare, these tools will empower you to take control of your health and your finances.

Chapter 7:

Telemedicine and Digital Healthcare Solutions

The rise of digital healthcare solutions has transformed the way we access and receive medical care. In particular, telemedicine has become a popular and cost-effective alternative to traditional in-person visits, offering patients a convenient way to consult with healthcare providers remotely. This chapter will explore how telemedicine, online pharmacies, and remote monitoring devices are reshaping healthcare, making it more accessible and affordable for patients. By understanding these technologies, you can take advantage of the savings and conveniences they provide.

7.1 Telemedicine: A Cost-Effective Alternative to Traditional Visits

Telemedicine refers to the use of technology, particularly video conferencing, to provide healthcare services remotely. Over the last decade, telemedicine has emerged as a cost-effective solution for both patients and healthcare providers. It allows individuals to consult with doctors, specialists, and other healthcare professionals from the comfort of their homes, reducing the need for in-person visits.

Cost Savings for Patients

One of the primary advantages of telemedicine is its ability to reduce healthcare costs. For routine consultations, telemedicine appointments are often cheaper than traditional in-office visits. Patients save not only on the consultation fees but also on transportation costs, time off work, and other expenses associated with visiting a clinic or hospital.

For example, a study by Health Affairs found that the average cost of a telemedicine visit is about $79, compared to $146 for an in-person visit to a doctor's office. For individuals with high-deductible insurance plans or those paying out-of-pocket, this price difference can add up to substantial savings over time.

Convenience and Accessibility

In addition to being cost-effective, telemedicine is also incredibly convenient, particularly for individuals living in rural or underserved areas. With telemedicine, patients no longer need to travel long distances to see specialists or access medical care. This improved accessibility can lead to earlier diagnosis and treatment, potentially preventing more serious health issues that could result in higher medical costs down the line.

Furthermore, telemedicine offers more flexible scheduling, allowing patients to book appointments outside of traditional office hours. This flexibility can be particularly beneficial for working professionals or caregivers who may have difficulty finding time for in-person visits.

Telemedicine for Mental Health

Telemedicine has also become a popular option for mental health services, including therapy and psychiatric consultations. The convenience and affordability of teletherapy sessions make it easier for individuals to access mental health care, which is often less expensive than traditional therapy sessions in a physical office. Many online platforms now offer counseling and therapy services at lower costs, providing accessible mental health care options.

7.2 Virtual Care vs. In-Person Care: Pros, Cons, and Cost Differences

While telemedicine offers many benefits, it is important to understand when virtual care is appropriate and when in-person care is necessary. Both options have their pros and cons, and the choice between them depends on the nature of the medical issue, personal preferences, and cost considerations.

Pros of Virtual Care

1. Cost Savings: As mentioned earlier, virtual care is generally less expensive than in-person care. Patients save on consultation fees, transportation, and other incidental costs.

2. Convenience: Virtual care eliminates the need to visit a healthcare facility, making it more convenient for patients with busy schedules or those living in remote areas.

3. Access to Specialists: Telemedicine allows patients to consult with specialists who may not be available in their local area. This can be particularly helpful for rare or complex medical conditions.

Cons of Virtual Care

1. Limited Physical Examination: While telemedicine is suitable for consultations, some medical conditions require a physical examination that can only be performed in person. For example, a doctor cannot perform a physical exam or diagnostic tests like bloodwork or imaging during a virtual visit.

2. Technical Issues: Virtual care relies on technology, and patients may encounter technical difficulties such as poor internet connection, making it challenging to communicate effectively with their healthcare provider.

When to Opt for In-Person Care

While telemedicine is ideal for routine consultations, follow-ups, and managing chronic conditions, there are certain situations where in-person care is necessary. For example:

- Emergency Situations: In case of emergencies such as heart attacks, strokes, or serious injuries, in-person care is essential.

- Complex Diagnostic Procedures: Some medical conditions require diagnostic tests, physical examinations, or procedures that can only be conducted in a clinical setting.

Ultimately, the choice between virtual and in-person care depends on the nature of the medical issue, with many patients opting for a combination of both to maximize convenience and minimize costs.

7.3 The Rise of Online Pharmacies: Convenience and Savings

Online pharmacies have become a popular alternative to traditional brick-and-mortar drugstores, offering a more convenient and often cheaper way to purchase medications. As more people seek ways to save on prescription drug costs, the rise of online pharmacies provides a valuable solution for both affordability and accessibility.

Convenience of Online Pharmacies

The convenience of online pharmacies is one of their most significant benefits. Patients can order their prescriptions from the comfort of their homes and have them delivered directly to their doorsteps. This is especially useful for individuals with mobility issues or those living in rural areas with limited access to pharmacies.

Cost Savings

Online pharmacies can offer significant cost savings on prescription medications. Many online platforms negotiate lower prices with pharmaceutical companies, passing the savings on to customers. Additionally, some online pharmacies provide generic medications at a fraction of the cost of brand-name drugs, helping patients further reduce their prescription drug expenses.

Subscription Services

Several online pharmacies now offer subscription services for medications that patients take regularly. These services often come with discounts for bulk orders or automatic refills, making it easier for patients to manage their prescriptions and save money in the long run.

Safety and Legitimacy Concerns

While online pharmacies offer many advantages, it is essential to ensure that you are purchasing medications from a legitimate and licensed pharmacy. There are numerous fraudulent websites that sell counterfeit or expired drugs, which can pose serious health risks. To avoid this, always verify that the online pharmacy is certified by the National Association of Boards of Pharmacy (NABP) or a similar regulatory body.

7.4 Remote Monitoring Devices: Reducing Doctor Visits and Costs

Remote monitoring devices are transforming how patients manage chronic conditions and monitor their health. These devices allow patients to track their vital signs and other health metrics from home, reducing the need for frequent doctor visits and hospitalizations.

How Remote Monitoring Devices Work

Remote monitoring devices are wearable or home-based technologies that track health data in real-time. Examples include:

- Blood pressure monitors for individuals with hypertension.
- Glucose monitors for patients with diabetes.
- Wearable heart monitors for those with cardiovascular conditions.

These devices transmit data directly to healthcare providers, allowing them to monitor the patient's condition remotely. If any abnormal readings are detected, the healthcare provider can intervene before the condition worsens, preventing the need for an in-person visit or hospitalization.

Cost Savings and Health Benefits

By allowing patients to manage chronic conditions from home, remote monitoring devices reduce the frequency of doctor visits and emergency room trips. This not only saves time and money but also improves health outcomes by enabling earlier intervention and better disease management. For example, individuals with diabetes who use continuous glucose monitors (CGMs) may experience fewer complications and hospitalizations, ultimately reducing their overall healthcare costs.

The Growing Market for Remote Monitoring Devices

The market for remote monitoring devices is expanding rapidly as more patients and healthcare providers recognize the benefits of these technologies. Many insurance companies are also starting to cover the cost of remote monitoring devices, further reducing the financial burden on patients.

In conclusion, telemedicine, online pharmacies, and remote monitoring devices are revolutionizing healthcare by making it more accessible, convenient, and cost-effective. By leveraging these digital healthcare solutions, you can take better control of your health while reducing your medical expenses. Understanding how and when to use these tools can lead to significant savings and improve the overall quality of your care.

Chapter 8: High-Deductible Health Plans (HDHPs)

High-Deductible Health Plans (HDHPs) are becoming more common in today's healthcare landscape as employers and insurers shift towards these cost-saving strategies. HDHPs offer lower monthly premiums, making them an attractive option for many individuals and families. However, they come with a trade-off: higher out-of-pocket costs before insurance coverage kicks in. This chapter will delve into what HDHPs are, their advantages and disadvantages, strategies to manage costs, and how to use Health Savings Accounts (HSAs) to offset these higher expenses.

8.1 Understanding High-Deductible Health Plans: Benefits and Risks

A High-Deductible Health Plan (HDHP) is a type of health insurance that has lower monthly premiums but higher deductibles than traditional health plans. This means that you'll pay more out-of-pocket for healthcare services before your insurance starts covering a portion of the costs. HDHPs are typically paired with Health Savings

Accounts (HSAs), which allow individuals to set aside pre-tax dollars to pay for qualifying medical expenses.

Key Features of HDHPs:

- Lower Monthly Premiums: One of the most attractive features of HDHPs is the lower premium costs. For individuals and families looking to save on their monthly health insurance payments, HDHPs can be a cost-effective option.
- Higher Deductibles: While the premiums are lower, HDHPs come with higher deductibles, meaning you must pay a larger amount out-of-pocket for medical services before your insurance coverage begins. For 2024, the IRS defines a high-deductible plan as one with a minimum deductible of $1,600 for an individual or $3,200 for a family.
- HSA Eligibility: Individuals enrolled in HDHPs are often eligible to open an HSA, which allows them to save money tax-free for medical expenses.

Benefits of HDHPs:

- Lower Premiums: The reduced cost of monthly premiums can lead to significant savings, especially for healthy individuals who rarely need medical care.
- Incentive for Preventive Care: Many HDHPs offer free or low-cost preventive care, such as annual check-ups and vaccinations, even before the deductible is met. This encourages individuals to take a proactive approach to their health.
- HSA Contributions: HDHPs are designed to be used in conjunction with HSAs, which provide tax benefits and help individuals save for future medical expenses.

Risks of HDHPs:

- High Out-of-Pocket Costs: The most significant risk of an HDHP is the higher out-of-pocket expenses. If you or a family member experiences a major health event, such as surgery or hospitalization, you could face substantial upfront costs before your insurance begins covering services.
- Financial Strain for Unplanned Healthcare: For individuals with unpredictable health needs, HDHPs can lead to financial strain. Without sufficient savings or an HSA, covering high deductibles can be challenging.
- Delay in Seeking Care: Some individuals may delay seeking care due to the high out-of-pocket costs associated with HDHPs, which can worsen health conditions and lead to more expensive treatments later on.

8.2 Managing Costs with HDHPs: Planning for Out-of-Pocket Expenses

When choosing an HDHP, one of the most critical considerations is planning for the out-of-pocket costs you'll incur before reaching your deductible. The key to successfully managing these expenses is being proactive and prepared. Below are strategies to help manage healthcare costs under an HDHP:

Understanding Your Deductible and Out-of-Pocket Maximum

The first step in managing your healthcare costs with an HDHP is understanding your plan's deductible and out-of-pocket maximum. The deductible is the amount you must pay before your insurance covers any expenses, while the out-of-pocket maximum is the most you'll have to pay in a year before your insurance covers 100% of the remaining costs.

Creating an Emergency Healthcare Fund

Since HDHPs require higher upfront payments for medical services, it's crucial to have an emergency healthcare fund in place. Ideally, this fund should be large enough to cover your deductible and out-of-pocket maximum. By setting aside money each month, you can avoid financial stress when unexpected healthcare expenses arise.

Utilizing Preventive Services

HDHPs often cover preventive care services at no cost to you, even before you meet your deductible. These services may include annual physicals, immunizations, cancer screenings, and other preventive measures. Taking advantage of these benefits can help you maintain your health and catch potential health issues early, which can prevent larger healthcare costs down the line.

Negotiating Medical Bills

Under an HDHP, you'll pay the full cost of many medical services until you reach your deductible. One way to manage these costs is by negotiating with healthcare providers. Many doctors and hospitals offer payment plans, sliding scales, or discounts for patients paying out-of-pocket. You can also ask for an itemized bill to ensure there are no errors or unnecessary charges.

8.3 Using HSAs to Offset High-Deductible Costs

Health Savings Accounts (HSAs) are one of the most valuable tools for individuals enrolled in HDHPs. These accounts allow you to save pre-tax dollars to pay for qualified medical expenses, helping you offset the costs associated with your high deductible. HSAs offer several financial advantages that make them a powerful tool for managing healthcare expenses.

Tax Advantages of HSAs

HSAs provide three significant tax benefits:

1. Contributions Are Tax-Deductible: Contributions made to an HSA reduce your taxable income, lowering the amount of taxes you owe.
2. Tax-Free Growth: The money in your HSA grows tax-free over time. Any interest or investment gains earned in the account are not subject to taxes.
3. Tax-Free Withdrawals: Withdrawals from your HSA are tax-free as long as they are used to pay for qualified medical expenses.

Maximizing HSA Contributions

For 2024, the IRS allows individuals to contribute up to $4,150 to their HSAs, while families can contribute up to $8,300. Individuals over the age of 55 can contribute an additional $1,000 as a "catch-up" contribution. To fully benefit from an HSA, it's a good idea to contribute the maximum allowed each year.

Using HSA Funds Wisely

HSAs can be used for a wide range of qualified medical expenses, including doctor's visits, prescription drugs, dental care, vision care, and more. Because HSA funds never expire, you can roll them over year after year, allowing you to build up a significant balance for future medical expenses. If you remain healthy and don't use the funds, they can also serve as a supplemental retirement savings account, as HSA funds can be withdrawn for any purpose without penalty after age 65 (though non-medical withdrawals will be subject to income tax).

Saving for Future Healthcare Needs

An HSA is not just for current medical expenses—it can also be used as a long-term savings tool. Many people use their HSAs to save for future healthcare needs, including retirement healthcare costs. Medical expenses are likely to increase as you age, so having a substantial balance in your HSA can help cover those future costs.

8.4 Budgeting for Healthcare with an HDHP

Since HDHPs require you to pay a larger portion of your healthcare expenses out-of-pocket, creating a healthcare budget is essential. Proper budgeting can help you prepare for routine medical expenses, as well as unexpected costs. Here's how to create a healthcare budget when enrolled in an HDHP:

Estimate Your Annual Healthcare Costs

The first step in budgeting for healthcare is estimating your expected annual healthcare costs. Consider your current health status, any ongoing medical treatments or prescriptions, and your family's healthcare needs. Include routine expenses like annual check-ups, dental cleanings, and prescription medications, as well as potential emergency or unexpected medical needs.

Factor in Your Deductible and Out-of-Pocket Maximum

When budgeting for healthcare under an HDHP, it's crucial to account for both your deductible and your out-of-pocket maximum. Plan to set aside enough money to cover these amounts, either in a separate savings account or through your HSA. If your plan has a high deductible, ensure that you're financially prepared to pay that amount in the event of a medical emergency.

Track Your Healthcare Spending

Throughout the year, keep track of your healthcare spending to ensure that you're staying within your budget. This can also help you identify areas where you may be able to cut costs, such as using generic medications or choosing less expensive providers. Tracking your spending also allows you to see how close you are to meeting your deductible and out-of-pocket maximum.

Review Your Plan Annually

Since healthcare needs change over time, it's important to review your HDHP and healthcare budget annually. During your employer's open enrollment period or when choosing a plan on the health insurance marketplace, evaluate whether your current HDHP still meets your needs. If you anticipate higher medical expenses in the coming year, you may want to consider switching to a different plan or increasing your HSA contributions.

In conclusion, High-Deductible Health Plans offer both benefits and risks. By understanding the specifics of your HDHP, utilizing an HSA, and carefully budgeting for healthcare expenses, you can navigate the financial challenges of these plans and make the most of their cost-saving potential. Proper planning and smart healthcare decisions will help you minimize out-of-pocket costs and ensure you're financially prepared for any medical expenses that arise.

Chapter 9:

Managing Chronic Illness and Long-Term Care Costs

Chronic illness and long-term care are major concerns for millions of individuals and their families, given the significant financial burden they can impose. Managing a chronic disease often requires ongoing treatment, prescription medications, and frequent doctor visits, all of which can lead to high medical expenses. Similarly, long-term care, particularly for aging individuals, can be financially overwhelming. In this chapter, we'll explore strategies to reduce the costs of managing chronic conditions, find affordable long-term care solutions, and tap into resources and programs that help alleviate the financial strain.

9.1 Strategies for Reducing Costs of Chronic Disease Management

Managing a chronic illness can be expensive, but there are several strategies to reduce the costs while ensuring you or your loved ones receive the necessary care.

Work with Healthcare Providers to Develop a Cost-Efficient Care Plan

Communication with healthcare providers is crucial when managing chronic illness. Ask your doctor about the most essential treatments and which interventions could be delayed or simplified without compromising health. Often, there are lower-cost alternatives to expensive medications or procedures that can be equally effective. Additionally, some healthcare providers offer financial assistance programs or payment plans for patients struggling to cover the cost of care.

Choose Generic Medications Over Brand-Name Drugs

Medications are often a significant component of chronic disease management. One of the most straightforward ways to cut costs is to switch to generic versions of prescribed drugs. Generic medications contain the same active ingredients as their brand-name counterparts but are often much less expensive. Be sure to ask your doctor if a generic option is available for any prescriptions.

Utilize Prescription Discount Programs

Prescription drug discount programs can offer significant savings, especially for those managing chronic conditions. Several websites, apps, and cards offer discounts on prescription medications, such as GoodRx and SingleCare. Many pharmacies also offer their own discount programs or allow patients to use manufacturer coupons, which can drastically reduce out-of-pocket costs.

Leverage Telemedicine for Routine Check-ups

Telemedicine can be a cost-effective option for routine check-ins and management of chronic illnesses. Virtual visits often cost less than in-person visits and can help patients avoid unnecessary emergency room or urgent care visits for manageable conditions. Many healthcare providers offer telemedicine options, especially for patients with chronic diseases like diabetes or hypertension, where regular monitoring is crucial.

Participate in Disease Management Programs

Many health insurance plans offer disease management programs designed to help patients manage chronic conditions. These programs provide educational resources, personalized health coaching, and regular check-ins to ensure that patients are following their care plans effectively. By participating in such programs, patients can often reduce the frequency of costly hospital visits or emergency care by staying on top of their condition.

9.2 Finding Affordable Long-Term Care and Elder Care Solutions

Long-term care costs can be a major financial burden for families, especially for those providing care to elderly loved ones. Fortunately, there are several ways to reduce the financial strain and find more affordable solutions for elder care.

Explore Home-Based Care Options

Home-based care can be a more affordable and comfortable option compared to nursing homes or assisted living facilities. Depending on the level of care needed, families can hire in-home care aides or home health nurses to assist with daily activities or medical needs. Additionally, many states have Medicaid waiver programs that provide financial assistance for home-based care, allowing individuals to remain in their homes rather than moving to a more expensive facility.

Look for Community-Based Services

Many communities offer low-cost or free services to help seniors with daily living activities. These services may include meal delivery, transportation to medical appointments, and adult day care programs. Community centers, religious organizations, and local government agencies often provide these services at reduced costs or on a sliding scale based on income.

Consider Long-Term Care Insurance

Long-term care insurance can help cover the costs of long-term care services, including nursing home care, assisted living, or home-based care. While long-term care insurance can be expensive, it is worth considering for individuals with chronic illnesses or those who expect to need significant care in the future. Purchasing a policy earlier in life, when rates are typically lower, can provide peace of mind and protect against the high costs of long-term care later on.

Medicaid for Long-Term Care

Medicaid is one of the largest payers of long-term care services in the United States. Individuals who meet Medicaid's income and asset eligibility criteria can qualify for nursing home care or home- and community-based services. Each state has its own guidelines for eligibility, so it's important to research the options available in your area. For individuals with limited financial resources, Medicaid can be an essential resource for accessing long-term care services.

9.3 Resources and Programs for Managing Ongoing Medical Needs

Various government programs, non-profits, and private organizations offer resources to help individuals with chronic conditions manage ongoing medical needs. Here are some of the key resources available:

Medicare for Chronic Care

Medicare provides several options for individuals managing chronic conditions. For example, Medicare Part D offers prescription drug coverage, which can help lower the costs of medications for chronic diseases. Medicare Advantage plans may also offer additional benefits, such as coordinated care or disease management programs, designed to assist individuals with chronic illnesses.

Non-Profit Assistance Programs

Many non-profit organizations provide financial assistance or services to individuals with chronic illnesses. Organizations such as the American Cancer Society, the American Heart Association, and the National Kidney Foundation offer various forms of support, including help with medical bills, transportation to medical appointments, and free or low-cost screenings.

Patient Assistance Programs from Pharmaceutical Companies

Many pharmaceutical companies offer patient assistance programs (PAPs) for individuals who cannot afford their medications. These programs provide free or discounted prescription drugs to eligible patients. Individuals with chronic conditions that require ongoing medication can apply for assistance through these programs by working with their healthcare provider or visiting the manufacturer's website.

Chronic Disease Management Grants

Some states and local governments provide grants or financial assistance programs to individuals managing chronic illnesses. These programs can help cover the costs of medical equipment, home modifications, or in-home care. Researching what's available in your state or municipality can uncover potential resources to ease the financial burden of ongoing care.

9.4 Planning for Medical Emergencies: How to Prepare Financially

While it's impossible to predict when a medical emergency will occur, planning for these unexpected events can help you manage the financial burden they may bring. Here are some strategies to prepare for medical emergencies:

Create an Emergency Healthcare Fund

Setting aside money in an emergency healthcare fund can help cover unexpected medical expenses that may arise from chronic illnesses or accidents. This fund should be separate from other savings and designated specifically for healthcare-related costs, such as hospital visits, medications, or emergency treatments. Aim to build up a fund that covers at least your insurance deductible and out-of-pocket maximum.

Know Your Insurance Coverage

Understanding what your health insurance covers in an emergency is crucial. Review your policy to know what services are included, such as ambulance rides, emergency room visits, and hospital stays. Also, familiarize yourself with your plan's network of providers, so you know which hospitals and emergency services you can access at lower costs.

Consider Supplemental Insurance

In addition to traditional health insurance, some individuals may benefit from supplemental insurance policies, such as accident or critical illness insurance. These policies provide cash payouts that can help cover out-of-pocket medical expenses in the event of an emergency. Supplemental insurance can be especially valuable for those managing chronic illnesses or facing high medical costs.

Review Advanced Directives and Power of Attorney

For individuals managing chronic conditions, having legal documents such as an advanced healthcare directive and a durable power of attorney can help ensure that medical decisions align with their preferences in the event of an emergency. These documents also allow a designated person to make financial and healthcare decisions on behalf of the individual if they are unable to do so themselves.

In conclusion, managing chronic illness and long-term care costs can be daunting, but there are many strategies, resources, and programs available to help reduce the financial strain. By taking advantage of cost-saving measures, government assistance, and proper financial planning, individuals and families can ensure they receive the care they need without sacrificing their financial stability.

Chapter 10: Conclusion and Next Steps

As we reach the end of this guide, it's essential to take a moment to reflect on the strategies, tools, and resources presented throughout the book. Managing healthcare costs, navigating insurance systems, and seeking affordable care can seem overwhelming at times, but by being proactive, informed, and strategic, it's possible to significantly reduce medical expenses while maintaining your health and well-being. This chapter will recap the key strategies discussed, emphasize the importance of making informed decisions about your health and finances, and offer additional resources for continued learning and support.

10.1 Recap of Key Strategies to Reduce Healthcare Costs

Throughout this book, we've explored numerous ways to manage and reduce healthcare costs without sacrificing the quality of care. Here's a quick summary of the key strategies that can help you lower your medical expenses:

- Understanding Your Medical Bills and Insurance: By decoding your medical bills and knowing what each charge represents, you can avoid unnecessary expenses and spot potential errors. Additionally, understanding your insurance policy—how premiums, deductibles, co-pays, and networks work—will help you choose the right plan for your needs and reduce out-of-pocket costs.

- Prescription Drug Costs: Prescription drug prices are rising, but strategies such as opting for generic medications, using prescription discount programs, and exploring therapeutic alternatives can help you save significantly. Online pharmacies and patient assistance programs can also provide cheaper alternatives to traditional purchasing methods.

- Utilizing Government and Non-Profit Programs: Medicare, Medicaid, and other government assistance programs offer support for those with high healthcare costs. Additionally, non-profit organizations and patient assistance programs from pharmaceutical companies provide resources and financial aid for managing chronic conditions and covering medical bills.

- Healthcare Savings Strategies: Leveraging Health Savings Accounts (HSAs) and Flexible Spending Accounts (FSAs) allows you to save money pre-tax for healthcare-related expenses. Additionally, shopping for affordable healthcare providers, community clinics, and low-cost medical procedures can reduce the burden of routine care.

- Becoming Your Own Healthcare Advocate: By asking the right questions, negotiating bills, and learning when to dispute charges, you can avoid overpaying for medical services. In certain situations, hiring a medical billing advocate can save you money by uncovering errors and negotiating lower fees.

- Telemedicine and Digital Healthcare Solutions: Telemedicine has emerged as a cost-effective alternative to traditional in-person visits. Virtual care, online pharmacies, and remote monitoring devices offer convenience and savings, particularly for routine care and managing chronic conditions.

- Managing High-Deductible Health Plans (HDHPs): If you have an HDHP, careful planning for out-of-pocket expenses is crucial. Using HSAs to offset costs and budgeting for healthcare expenses can help you manage the risks and benefits of these plans.

- Chronic Illness and Long-Term Care Costs: For individuals managing chronic illnesses, finding affordable long-term care, leveraging resources such as community services, and using prescription discount programs are essential. Planning for emergencies and creating an emergency healthcare fund ensures you're financially prepared for unexpected medical needs.

These strategies form the foundation for reducing healthcare costs and ensuring that your medical care aligns with your financial goals. While not every method may apply to your situation, combining the right approaches can lead to significant savings and better management of healthcare expenses.

10.2 Making Informed Decisions About Your Health and Finances

One of the most important takeaways from this book is the value of making informed decisions about both your health and finances. Healthcare costs can be unpredictable, and without careful planning, they can quickly overwhelm your budget. However, by staying informed, you can make proactive choices that prevent medical expenses from spiraling out of control.

Here are some final tips to help you make smarter decisions:

- Research Before Making Healthcare Decisions: Whether you're choosing an insurance plan, undergoing a medical procedure, or selecting a healthcare provider, take the time to thoroughly research your options. Compare costs, understand your coverage, and ask for detailed explanations from healthcare providers when needed. Making informed decisions will reduce the risk of unexpected expenses.

- Be Proactive About Preventive Care: Investing in preventive care, such as annual check-ups, screenings, and vaccinations, can help you catch health issues early and avoid more expensive treatments down the road. Preventive care often costs less and is sometimes covered by insurance, making it a smart investment for long-term health.

- Create a Healthcare Budget: It's important to plan for medical expenses just as you would for other aspects of your financial life. Budget for routine healthcare costs, such as co-pays, prescriptions, and insurance premiums, and set aside savings for unexpected medical bills. If you have an HDHP, make sure you're prepared for the out-of-pocket costs by contributing regularly to an HSA.

- Know Your Legal Rights: As a patient, you have certain rights when it comes to your healthcare, including the right to dispute medical bills and receive clear explanations of your charges. Don't hesitate to challenge incorrect or excessive charges, and if necessary, seek the help of a medical billing advocate or legal professional to resolve disputes.

- Continuously Evaluate Your Healthcare Needs: As your health or financial situation changes, your healthcare needs may evolve. Periodically review your insurance coverage, prescription medication needs, and healthcare providers to ensure you're still getting the best value for your money. Adjusting your healthcare strategies in response to changing circumstances can help you stay financially stable.

10.3 Additional Resources for Continued Learning and Assistance

Navigating the complex world of healthcare and medical costs is an ongoing process. To help you stay informed and continue saving on healthcare, here are some additional resources you can explore:

- Government Websites:

  • [Healthcare.gov](https://www.healthcare.gov/): Provides information on health insurance options, eligibility, and enrollment for the Health Insurance Marketplace.
  • [Medicare.gov](https://www.medicare.gov/): Offers comprehensive details about Medicare, including coverage options, costs, and how to apply.
  • [Medicaid.gov](https://www.medicaid.gov/): Learn about Medicaid eligibility, benefits, and state-specific programs that can help with healthcare costs.

- Non-Profit Organizations:

  • [The Patient Advocate Foundation](https://www.patientadvocate.org/): Provides assistance with medical billing, insurance issues, and accessing healthcare for individuals with chronic conditions.
  • [NeedyMeds](https://www.needymeds.org/): A non-profit that helps people find patient assistance programs, discounted prescriptions, and other forms of financial assistance for medical expenses.

- Prescription Drug Savings:

- [GoodRx](https://www.goodrx.com/): Offers coupons and discounts for prescription medications, helping individuals save on their prescriptions at various pharmacies.
- [SingleCare](https://www.singlecare.com/): Provides similar savings on prescriptions, offering free discount cards and access to lower-cost medication options.

- Telemedicine and Virtual Healthcare:

- [Teladoc](https://www.teladoc.com/): A telemedicine platform that allows patients to consult with doctors remotely, often at a lower cost than traditional in-person visits.
- [MDLIVE](https://www.mdlive.com/): Another popular telehealth platform offering virtual consultations for a range of medical issues.

- Healthcare Financial Assistance:

- [National Patient Advocate Foundation](https://www.npaf.org/): Advocates for affordable healthcare and provides resources for individuals struggling with medical bills.
- [HealthWell Foundation](https://www.healthwellfoundation.org/): Offers financial assistance to patients with chronic or life-altering conditions to help cover medical costs.

By continuing to educate yourself, seek out resources, and explore assistance programs, you can take control of your healthcare expenses and ensure that you receive the care you need without putting your financial well-being at risk.

In conclusion, managing healthcare costs is not a one-time effort but a continuous process that requires awareness, advocacy, and planning. The strategies outlined in this book will empower you to make informed decisions about your health, reduce your medical expenses, and navigate the complex healthcare system more effectively. With the right knowledge and resources, you can protect both your health and your financial future.

References

1. Centers for Medicare & Medicaid Services (CMS). (2023). Medicare & You 2023. Available at: https://www.medicare.gov

2. GoodRx. (2023). Prescription Drug Discounts. Available at: https://www.goodrx.com

3. Kaiser Family Foundation (KFF). (2023). Health Insurance Marketplace Calculator. Available at: https://www.kff.org

4. National Patient Advocate Foundation. (2023). Healthcare Financial Assistance Programs. Available at: https://www.patientadvocate.org

5. HealthWell Foundation. (2023). Chronic Disease Financial Assistance Programs. Available at: https://www.healthwellfoundation.org

6. NeedyMeds. (2023). Find Prescription Assistance Programs. Available at: https://www.needymeds.org

7. Patient Advocate Foundation. (2023). Patient Services for Medical Debt and Financial Aid. Available at: https://www.patientadvocate.org

8. SingleCare. (2023). Prescription Savings Card. Available at:
https://www.singlecare.com

9. Teladoc. (2023). Telemedicine Services. Available at:
https://www.teladoc.com

10. The Commonwealth Fund. (2023). Health Insurance and Healthcare Cost Trends
in the U.S. Available at:
https://www.commonwealthfund.org

11. U.S. Department of Health and Human Services (HHS). (2023). Understanding
Medicaid Eligibility and Benefits. Available at:
https://www.medicaid.gov

100

Author's Note

As someone who has witnessed firsthand the financial strain that high medical costs can impose on individuals and families, I felt compelled to write this book to provide actionable strategies and resources to help you navigate the complicated world of healthcare expenses.

Healthcare is a fundamental right, yet for many, the costs associated with it create overwhelming financial burdens. Through this book, my hope is that you will feel empowered and equipped with the knowledge to make informed decisions, reduce your medical expenses, and advocate for yourself in every step of your healthcare journey.

I encourage you to seek out the resources and assistance programs mentioned here, and to remember that managing healthcare costs is not a journey you need to take alone. There are numerous organizations, tools, and strategies available to help you minimize expenses while ensuring you receive the care you need.

It is my sincere wish that this book serves as a valuable guide, offering practical advice that you can apply to your own healthcare situation. Thank you for allowing me to accompany you on this path toward financial wellness and better healthcare management.

Take care of yourself and your health—both physically and financially.

With warm regards,

Oluchi Ike

103